The Safety Muscles Guide

Your Guide to Relieving Back, Neck, Hip
and Shoulder Pain by Balancing Your
Posture at Home or in the Gym

Allison Ishman

**This guide is not intended to be a replacement for medical diagnosis or advice.
Always consult your doctor before beginning any exercise regimen.**

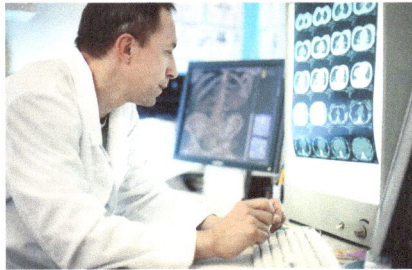

Table of Contents

THESE ARE THE
7 SAFETY MUSCLES

What Are Safety Muscles?

Safety muscles are the small postural muscles used to balance your muscle strength, improve your posture, and reduce risk of injury and common pain problems like neck or back pain, hamstring or groin tears, rotator cuff pain, and related shoulder and hip problems. The safety muscles balance the muscles you normally use in daily activities. The wisdom of safety muscle strengthening is that establishing better muscle balance allows you to more easily sit, stand, and do activities with better posture and less pain, and can reduce risk of injury. This is the "safety net" of muscles.

When I was in my 20's, I used to help my friends move, and would always do my safety muscles the day before I helped with the move. I never got sore if I did that. When I was seeing 6-8 patients a day in my clinic and felt a headache coming on or had a stiff back or neck, I did my safety muscle strengthening to immediately reduce the pressure of a headache or to balance my tight neck or back muscles. Over the years I shared this with my patients. Today, I am sharing this insight with you. This is a maintenance plan for the body. This is the little black book of tricks to keep your body humming when it's threatening to keep you from what you planned to do today! You have the 6 muscle group keys to better health in your hands right now.

Balanced strength around your joints and a tendency toward good posture has additional benefits, such as relief from tension and muscle pain, improved productivity, increased sports performance, and reduced risk of injury to muscles, tendons and joints. If you don't believe me, just try it for yourself. It takes about two weeks to take these weak muscle groups from zero to noticeable tone, and get out of the old, creaky body that may have inspired you to read this book at all!

Physically, the safety muscles include the small muscles that stabilize your shoulders and your hips. The areas we will focus on are lower shoulders, abdominals, and thigh muscles. These neglected areas are the key to balance in the body.

What difference does good posture make?

Most people think of walking with a book on your head, or of your mother telling you to sit up straight when they think of posture. These are interesting guidelines for looking good. We can even find scientists who study how good posture affects depression, self-esteem, positive outlook and other emotions. Studies about people-related jobs such as sales or marketing evaluate how posture is a reflection of your willingness to buy, how open your are to influence, and when you are really saying no to a sales pitch.

I am concerned with posture here as it relates to your ability to:

1. Stay strong, so you can do whatever activities you want to do, such as travel, go to events, and enjoy playing with friends and children
2. Perform activities in your life without pain and discomfort during or afterward
3. Feel healthy and be *willing to participate* in achieving your fitness goals as well as being a part of active social groups. If everyone is taking a walk or a hike, you should be able to go too!

In this guide, when I talk about evening out muscle tone or strength, I am referring to having balanced strength or muscle tone. *Balanced* or *even* strength gives you better protection of joints, reduced wear and tear on soft tissues in the body, and a higher energy level. When your muscles are in balance, you are not using up your chemical energy maintaining tension in muscles you rely on for posture.

With a healthy posture, you *will* look better. However, you will also *feel better* and *stay healthier*. So, in this situation I am not your mother – I'm your health care professional telling you to sit up straight, and giving you the information you need to do that more easily and naturally.

Why Call These Safety Muscles?

Too many people get injured when starting a strength-training program, or develop recurring and annoying pain or tension in their body due to muscle imbalances. I see this all the time in my clinical therapy and fitness work. Sometimes the pain comes and goes, and people begin to just tolerate it. This can range from hand or shoulder pain to back pain, or even menstrual cramps. Other times people will accept constant tension as part of life, such as tension in the neck and back, or a calf or hamstring that is always tight, is prone to tears, or herniates.

What hurts on different people always varies, as we are all doing different things with differently shaped bodies, differing genes and unique nutritional habits. But over the years, I began to see a pattern of the most commonly weak postural muscles.

These exercises balance the vast majority of postural problems that cause pain and nagging tightness, leave you prone to repetitive stress or sports injuries, make you slump and sag, and contribute to making you feel tired and sluggish. This is your guide to balancing the most common tight muscles in your body with the typically weak muscles that oppose or balance them.

Why are there commonly weak postural muscles?

Why are these typical weak muscles weak? The answer is because we don't use them. Let's consider our overall activities and how they affect our postural muscles.

Our tasks today seem to be relatively similar. We sit, stand, walk, run, ride bikes, carry things, and lean over. We also pick things up from the floor or shelf. As a whole, that's about it. Of course there are also less common actions such as slipping, falling or occasional heavy lifting. We will talk about the common actions first, and the atypical actions at the end. Let's dig in!

Sitting – Back and Abdominals

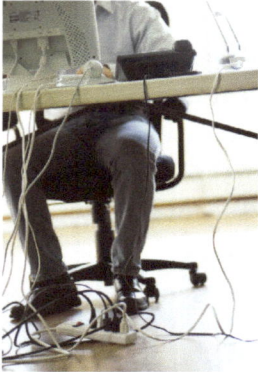

People today do a good amount of sitting. We sit at a desk, in a car, at a table, or on a couch. Sitting in chairs allows us to be upright without using our midsection much for stabilization. If we lean, we don't require very much abdominal strength to stay upright. So, as people sit forward on chairs, or slump in a chair, they don't use muscles evenly.

Even worse, if you sit in the chair and don't use the back support, your back muscles are always contracting to hold you up. So, your back muscles get tighter as you neglect to use your abdominals.

When sitting, with abdominal muscles getting little activity, we start to use muscles in our arms and legs for more motions. Our *weak abdominals* don't activate when we get up and down from chairs, and don't bother to wake up and help us when we climb stairs later in the day, since they've been at rest all along. With the increasing popularity of "core training", people are beginning to learn that stronger midsections lead to less wear and tear on the muscles of the legs and arms, and help the body work as a unit. So, our first exercise below is for the abdominal muscles.

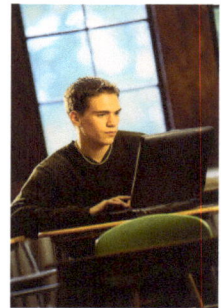

Sitting and Looking – Neck and Shoulders

Anytime we sit and focus on a computer or a book, on the road, at a classroom, boardroom, or jury of people, we keep our heads in fixated positions. There are not active times, and increasingly we find ourselves doing these tasks for hours on end. These stabilizing positions we are in so often reduce circulation in the neck and shoulders, and give us a tendency to bring our heads slightly forward as we focus.

Balancing motions such as overhead lifting and rowing are not part of our usual routines. Yet, these motions are the ones that build balance our shoulders by strengthening the small outside shoulder muscles. So, the first muscles I include below are designed to balance the shoulders, and reduce strain and tightness on the muscles of our neck and shoulders.

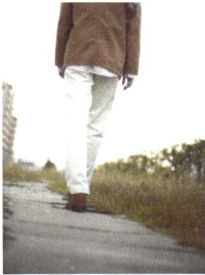

Standing, Walking and Running – Legs and Feet

Perhaps the most common activities after sitting are standing, walking, and running. We stand in lines, to speak or teach, to cook and to dress and do chores at home or work. We walk and run for transportation or exercise.

Are you weak?

All of these actions rely on leg muscles and tendons. Since tendons are thicker, more fibrous tissues in the body, we tend to rely on them especially when our muscles are not strong enough for the activities we do. So, if you are in a weaker state, you are probably using more tendons.

The most commonly stressed tendons from standing, walking and running with weak leg muscles are the iliotibial band (or ITB) tendon on whole outer thigh and hip, the upper hip flexors, inner thigh tendons by the pelvis, and in the Achilles tendon of the calf. The bottoms of the feet also tend to get tight from standing, walking and running frequently. This tissue on the bottoms of the feet we are concerned with is called the plantar fascia. We will refer to these commonly tight areas of the body in the following sections, as we balance the tension in the body.

Are you strong?

If you are an active person who has strong leg muscles, the next most important issue is the balance of strength between the front and back of your thighs, and between the inner and outer thighs. Usually, the lower 6 inches or so of your Hamstring (found on the back of the thigh) is tighter and stronger than the upper Hamstring. Conversely, the lower 6 inches or so of the front of the thigh is usually weaker muscle, with the tighter area being up by the top of the legs. These front muscles are called Quadriceps. So, they don't evenly balance one another in many active people.

With regard to inner and outer thighs, the inner thigh has a tendency to be tight by the pelvis, and weak by the knee. The outer thigh tends to be tight altogether, as this strong tendon is relied upon for holding you upright and moving about. Evening the tension here can have an impact on all of the related muscles, as is detailed later under the inner thigh exercise.

Lifting from shelves and floors, Carrying kids, bags and boxes.

When we lift, we usually pick up a thing or a child from the floor or from a shelf. With our already weak abdominal muscles, we use primarily chest and bicep muscles in the upper body, and our backs rather than our legs. Mindfulness of your posture can help, but actual strength in your safety muscles can enable you to do these actions with more fluid, less straining effort.

We carry bags on our shoulders with straps, and boxes with our arms, chest and backs most often. This still leaves out the abdominals, outside shoulder muscles, and legs. Heavy items use our legs, but most of us don't carry heavy items on a grade, which is the motion that gives us a little better natural postural balance. .

These actions are actually balanced by all seven Safety Muscles below, as they involve the arms, hips, and legs.

Balancing tight muscles with weak muscles.

After years of helping people balance overtight muscles and opposing weak muscles, I developed a program to reduce injury and pain by strengthening the weakest postural muscles first. I know that "core strength" is popular these days, and these exercises do also strengthen the core. But, they also balance muscles in the shoulders and hips that often get ignored. Over time, they have come to be known as "Safety Muscles".

Why strengthen Safety Muscles?

Safety First! I am always emphasizing the benefits of a safe strength-training program. One of the best ways to prevent injury is to strengthen weak muscles to even the tension from over-tight areas. Balance posture first for safety, then get stronger. Before doing strength training in a general or weight-loss oriented strength training program, you can simply start with 1-2 weeks of strengthening safety muscles, or at least include them with the other exercises you are doing. Taking the 10 or 15 minutes needed for Safety Muscle strengthening enables you to balance your body to reduce injury and gain control over areas that may be uncomfortably tight or painful.

The muscles that are already used every day are more prone to injury when strength training or working out if the opposing muscles are weak. This program is designed to strengthen your weak postural muscles first.

Because of the high risk of injury involved in beginning any new, rigorous, or repeated activity, I strongly advocate that everyone strengthen 7 core Safety Muscles. Strength in these muscles especially benefits people who are over-active, under-active, under high-stress, or doing a repetitive-motion activities.

When do I start doing Safety Muscle strengthening, and when do I start doing additional strength training exercises?

I recommend building Safety Muscles before strengthening major muscles used for weight loss, power, or just to look good is an outstanding approach to staying injury-free and feeling better, stronger, and having a smooth strength training progression. Safety Muscle strength is incredibly effective at preventing injury, helping you to recover from an injury, increasing your daily activity or sports performance, improving a person's ability to be more athletically aggressive, and reducing stress.

Strength training without building small core muscles first is somewhat risky; you never know what muscle you may pull or which joint may suffer from imbalanced muscle strength. Therefore, before you go out there and hit the leg presses, chest flys, bench presses, and calf machines, I recommend 1-3 weeks (2 weeks average) of strengthening Safety Muscles. Then watch your performance improve progressively as you stay injury free and happy!

These are the
7 Safety Muscles

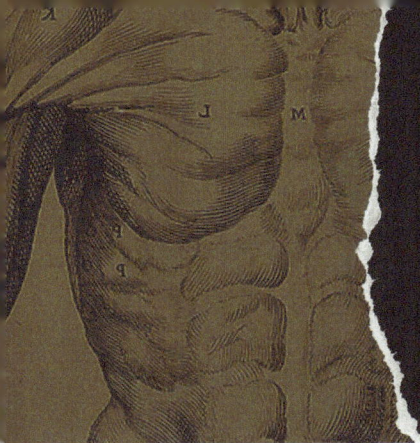

1
Abdominals

I prefer abdominal exercises that use the transverse abdominal muscle. The transverse abdominal is the deepest of the abdominal muscles, and is primarily responsible for stabilization and protection of the organs. However, it is also the most powerful way to unload the groin and hip flexors, and helps to balance the muscle and connective tissue load from activities such as standing, walking, running, and even sitting.

Half Rollback

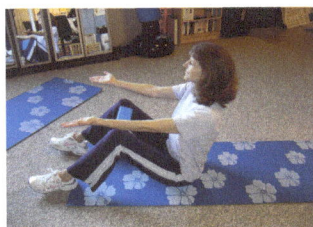

The first exercise I recommend is called the half rollback. It's a simple Pilates exercise, and starts in a seated position, feet on the floor and knees bent. To start, you will want something held stable between the knees, which activates the inner thigh muscles. Here I am showing a yoga block, but you can also use a Pilates ring, Pilates ball, kickball or a kids ball (something soft works best). You can even use a dictionary, if you're in a pinch. Palms face the ceiling. Inhale first to prepare, and as you exhale slowly roll back to a 45-degree position. Inhale holding that position, and as you exhale you return to an upright sitting position. It sounds simple,

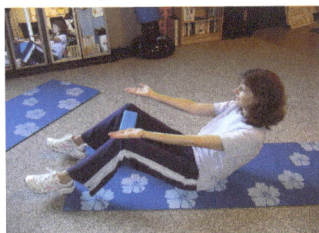

1

and it actually is simple. But, it requires stabilization from the transverse abdominal, and doing 8 repetitions in two sets 3 days per week will help to stabilize your transverse abdominal and give you the targeted core strength that unloads those postural imbalances, including relief for hip flexors and area leg muscles.

Why Strengthen Transverse Abdominal?

Strengthen abdominal muscle to prevent back pain and reduce back tension, and to reduce the load put on your groin / hip flexor muscles. Many adults that do not strengthen quadriceps, hamstrings, and inner thighs regularly, as well as stretch the muscles around the hips each week, carry a great deal of their upper body weight and the weight of bags, books, and other items they carry – with their hip flexor muscles. For more information about balance surrounding the hips, read my article titled "My Hips are Doing What?" at www.ibodycare.com. Strong abdominals look great as well – an added bonus for your self-esteem.

What Strengthening Transverse Abdominal Balances:

Improved abdominal strength takes pressure off of the psoas (groin) muscles, balances the tension in your back, and reduces the load of daily activities on your hips, chest. Through a series of structural and fascial lines in the body, abdominal strength reduces strain in your neck and all the way down to your feet. No kidding.

Transverse Abdominal Technical Muscle Balancing Information:

This exercise will strengthen abdominal muscles, therefore assisting with the release of hip flexors, and secondarily the iliotibial band (outer thigh). The common hip flexor muscle group that soft-tissue therapists are so often struggling to release in clients with pain is called the iliopsoas (il-ee-oh-so-as). Other common hip flexors you are unloading with this exercise are called the pectineus, tensor fascia latae (TFL), sartorius, adductor longus (an inner thigh muscle) and rectus femoris (the topmost quadricep).

Lower Butt (Glutes)

The exercises I like best for lower butt or gluteal muscles are kickbacks and T's. They are detailed here separately, starting with kickbacks. Kickbacks are easier for most people starting out, so we will begin with these.

Kickbacks

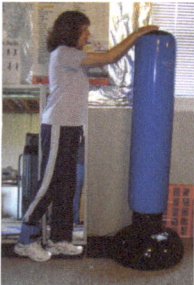

The kick back can be performed with or without ankle weight or using a cable with stacked weight. It can also be effective with no weight, depending on your strength level.

Start standing with one foot behind you and your toe toward the floor. Using lower butt, raise the leg behind you, hold and return.

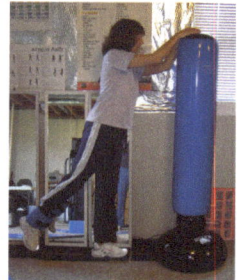

Do two sets of 10 repetitions 1-3 times per week.

Why Strengthen Lower Gluteals / Butt?

Strengthen the lower gluteus muscles to reduce the load on your hips and low back, reduce Hamstring stress, and to reduce load on groin and hip flexor muscles. A butt that doesn't sag also looks and feels more attractive, which is another added bonus for your self-esteem!

What Strengthening Lower Gluteals / Butt Does

Strengthening LOWER butt muscles reduces tension on the upper hip tendons that attach on the pelvis in the low back area. The flat, rubber-band-like connective tissues from the butt area also wrap up into the middle back and around to the abdomen and hip flexors, so this exercise can have an impact on low back pain. Lower butt strength also balances commonly found tension the groin and the upper sections of the thighs.

Lower Gluteals / Butt Technical Muscle Balancing Information:

Activities that strengthen gluteal muscle tend to take pressure off of the Sacroiliac joint at the base of the low back, and unload tension in iliopsoas, tensor fascia latae (TFL) and pectineus. Lower gluteal muscles also enable better postural stances, which can secondarily take tension off of ITB and the central hamstring tendon. Another secondary benefit is unloading of tension in the paraspinal group, as the fascia and strong muscle fibers in the back reduce the postural stabilization requirements of the paraspinals.

Another interesting relationship is that lower gluteal strength can unload blockage in the bladder meridian, which follows central Hamstring tension, sacral attachments, and paraspinals. This can have a significant impact on stress, as bladder meridian is associated with anxiety and controls other meridians that are heavily associated with stress in the body. Bladder meridian controls triplewarmer, which is responsible for safety and pleasing others. With the demanding lifestyles many professionals and parents live today, these are commonly stressed meridians. For more information about meridians, try using your favorite search engine and type in meridians. There is a wealth of information available online.

T's (Alternate Gluteal / Butt / More Challenging)

This exercise also builds the lower butt. I often have clients tell me it releases constipation as well. It is a little more challenging than the kickback, and can be made even more challenging when you add ankle weights. I suggest starting with no weight at first, just to get comfortable with the form. Add weight as the exercise feels easier, working your way up to 10 or even 20 pounds for stronger people.

Start on hands and knees as pictured. The focus here is to keep the hips VERY stable, and not to allow them to wiggle out of position. This means that you should not allow your spine to sidebend as your leg moves. Concentrate on aligning your spine with your hips and not bending the spine as you move. The movements here are small – only about 10-15 degrees. These are NOT intended to be large movements, as you cannot keep your hips stable and your spine from bending if your movement is too big.

Start Center

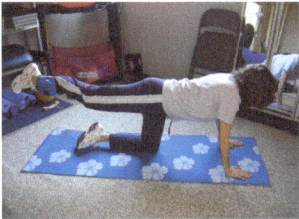

High (15 degrees)

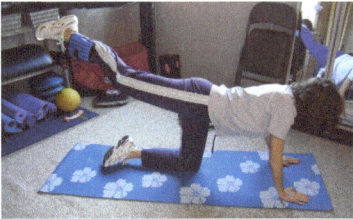

Center

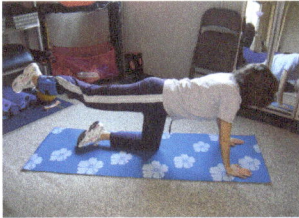

Out

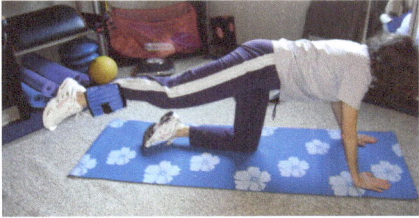

Center

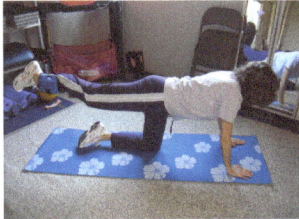

In

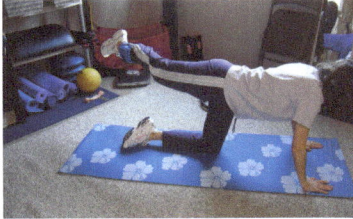

Center

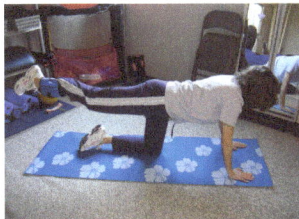

Tuck

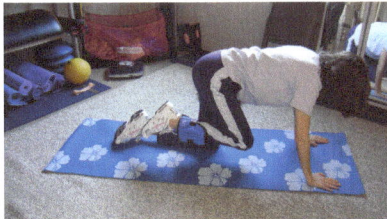

Repeat 6-10 times, resting when you are tired so that you use good form. Do two sets.

3

Inner Thigh

T his exercise is a common one, and is called an inner thigh leg raise. It is pictured below with ankle weight, but can be done without weight when first starting out. To begin, lay on one side with your upper body resting on your elbow. The inner thigh and arch of the foot should face the ceiling, and will stay facing the ceiling throughout the exercise. Inhale to prepare, and as you exhale you will raise your lower leg about halfway to the knee of the bent leg behind it. As you get stronger, you can lift up to the height of the back leg. When adding weight, start with 1-2 pounds, and make sure you're challenged but in control for 2 sets of 10 repetitions. Rest as needed, so you can maintain good form. Stronger people may progress to 10 or even 20 pounds over time.

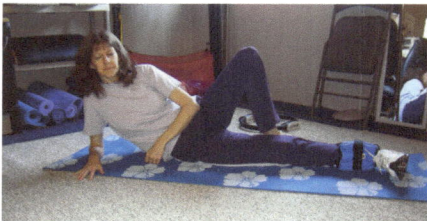

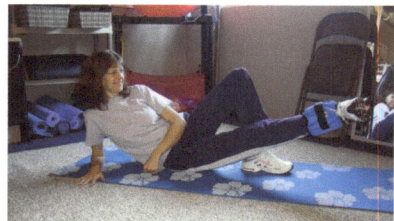

Why Strengthen Inner Thigh?

Strengthen the inner thigh to reduce the load on your iliotibial band (strong outer thigh tendon) and iliopsoas (groin). The ITB is a major weight bearing and high activity area – it carries a lot of the load. This is an overall stability muscle, and many people report that they feel more stable, stronger and better balanced when they do this exercise. Inner thighs are a large muscle group, and good strength here can give you the balance you need to have more power when walking, running, cycling, swimming, or doing any other sporting activity. Strength in this area will also reduce your recovery requirements following workouts, and reduce risk of injury in the legs from endurance and impact sports.

What Strengthening Inner Thigh Balances

Inner thigh strength balances the thick outer thigh tendon, which often gets very tight when you're active. It also gives much needed support to the knees for both active and less active people. Finally, it takes tension off of the hip flexor muscle attachments found at the very top of the inner thigh. Lessening tension on those upper inner thigh attachments helps you to keep your hips level, resulting in less back pain and tension. You may also feel relief from tension in the calves from strengthening inner thigh muscles.

Inner Thigh Technical Muscle Balancing Information:

The above exercise directly balances tightness found in the iliotibial band. It evens the compensatory tension that often arises in hip flexors, especially iliopsoas. Inner thigh strength assists in maintaining a strong lower quadricep and strong transverse abdominal groups, simply due to the close proximity and natural tendency of the body to use these structures for load bearing.

Secondary compensating muscles may also relax from postural compensation patterns after strengthening inner thigh muscles, including gastrocnemius, soleus, the peroneal group, anterior tibialis, the paraspinal muscle group, and the quadriceps.

*A Note About Using Inner Thigh Strengthening Equipment

I am not a big fan of circuit training equipment for the inner thigh. Since our focus is on the lower section of the inner thigh, and the tightest area of the inner thigh is already at the top, I don't like the pad usually used for inner thigh machines. Since the pad presses against the lower section of the inner thighs, it discourages the development of strength in the lower areas. These machines primarily build the upper section of the inner thigh, which is already over-tight in most people. If you use equipment at your gym and opt not to use ankle weight, I suggest using the large cable crossover machine, which has a weight stack at either end. You can use an ankle cuff with this weight stack and avoid a pad pressing on your lower inner thigh. This is an equally good way to get balanced hips with inner thigh strengthening, and is considered as good as the floor exercise pictured above.

Lower Quadriceps

Quadricep extensions shown below are common exercises in many strength programs. However, our focus is on where in the quad extension you put your emphasis. The most important part of the quad extension is the last 15 degrees, which uses primarily the inside knee attachments. For an overall guideline, however, we are going to focus on the last 45 degrees of a quad extension. This concentrates on the section of the quadriceps just above the knee, and helps to balance the lower section of the hamstring muscles in the back of the leg.

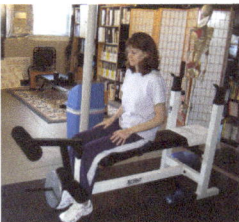

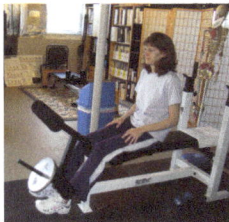

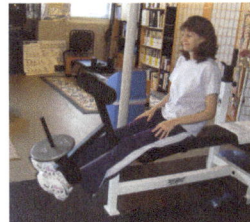

* Exercise can also be performed with ankle weights on a high stool, bench or bed.

Why Strengthen Lower Quadriceps?

The lower section of the quadriceps is the front of the thigh. Building strength here gives greater support to the knee, but most importantly takes pressure off of the hip flexors that become chronically tight. Also, strength in lower quads gives you more power for stairs and hills, allowing you to have better control. Focus on the last 45 degrees of a leg extension to strengthen here.

What Strengthening Lower Quadriceps Balances:

This balances and takes pressure off of the hip flexors and hamstrings. These strong leg muscles need balance to keep your hips from tilting out of a normal position.

Lower Quadriceps Technical Muscle Balancing Information:

Lower quadriceps are usually responsible for unloading postural and activity-based hypertonicity in hamstring fibers found just proximal to the knee. As hamstrings usually fire often in walking and running activities, and remain in a short position while sitting, these hamstring fibers are more often hypertonic than not. Stronger proximal quadriceps muscle will help posturally balance this tension and restore a protective muscle balance to support knee joints. In addition, lower quadriceps strength will reduce the load on upper quadriceps and hip flexor fibers that are often found in patients with weak safety muscles.

5
Teres

There are actually two muscles here we are focusing on, which are called teres major and teres minor. They perform the same actions at the shoulder that the latissimus dorsi or "lat muscle" does for the back and arms. These muscles help you pull back and down. This is the motion you would use bringing a box down from a high shelf, or a bale of hay from a stack of hay. Since we many people do this motion very rarely, these muscles tend to get weak and most people find this exercise challenging at first.

While this exercise it often not intuitive to many people, these small muscles are known for reducing neck tension and strain, as well as reducing or eliminating headaches. These muscles also balance midback tension.

Starting in a scarecrow position, inhale to prepare. Exhale and tuck your shoulders back and in, with the weights ending up next to your butt. The goal here is to use the muscles in the armpit area, which begin at the outside border of your shoulder blade and attach to the arm.

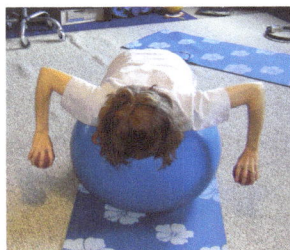

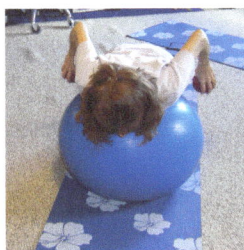

Why Strengthen Teres Muscles?

Strength and tone in teres muscles help balance tight necks and mid-backs. For some people, strengthening this muscle directly gets rid of a headache. So you can strengthen these outer shoulder muscles to reduce headaches and neck pain, forearm strain and carpal tunnel like conditions.

What Strengthening the Teres Muscle Group Balances:

This evens out the stress in muscles of the neck, back, and chest.

Teres Muscle Group Technical Balancing Information:

Teres muscle group strength unloads hypertonicity in scalenes, sternocleidomastoid (SCM), trapezius, rhomboids major and minor, levator scapulae, pectoralis major and pectoralis minor, and even splenius capiti muscles (secondarily).

6

Rotator Cuff

To strengthen the muscles of the shoulder blade area, start with your elbows bent 90 degrees and tuck them to the waist. Breathe in, and as you exhale, rotate at the shoulder and bring the weights away from your waist. I use an "eagle fly" prompt to help my clients remember this movement. You may do this exercise one side at a time, or combine them for two at a time to improve your efficiency. Start with 1 or two pound oxygen balls like they are shown here, and progress to 5 or 8 pounds maximum. This is challenging!

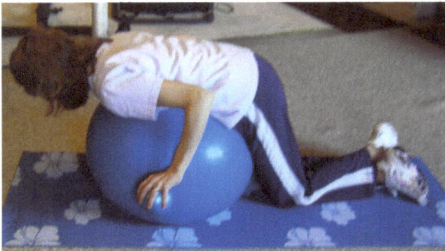

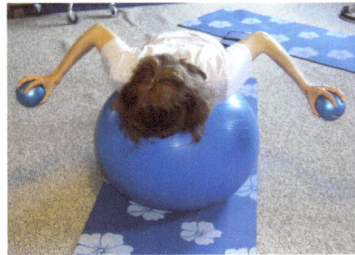

Why Strengthen Rotator Cuff Muscles?

Rotator cuff muscles typically get weak because we don't use them, like the teres muscles. Often people tear them because the tendons get so tight and the muscle belly is so weak and flabby that they just pull right apart. In this case, a little strengthening can go a long way to take pressure off of the neck and upper back. Again, we are strengthening the lower shoulder to reduce headaches and neck pain, forearm strain and carpal tunnel like conditions.

What Strengthening Rotator Cuff Muscles Balances:

This evens out the stress in muscles of the neck, back, and chest.

Technical Rotator Cuff Muscle Balancing Information:

The rotator cuff muscles include fours muscles, sometimes called SITS muscles. They are subscapularis, infraspinatus, teres minor, and supraspinatus. They attach on the greater tubercle of the humerus, thereby providing lateral stability to the scapula bones. Directly, these SITS fibers provide balancing muscle tone to rhomboids major and minor, levator scapula, and trapezius fibers. Secondarily, as fascial tension spreads, strength in the rotator cuff muscles balances flexors in the torso, including pectoralis fibers, biceps femoris, and even SCM and scalenes.

7

Posterior Deltoid

To strengthen posterior deltoid, commonly referred to as "rear delt", you will start on a bench or ball facing the floor, with light weights in each hand. Here, our model is using a 2-pound weight. Elbows are extended and weights rest on the floor, palms facing down toward the floor. Inhale to prepare, and as you exhale raise your arms to be level with your shoulders. Lower, and repeat 8-10 times, two sets. Progress in weight to 5 pounds over time, with the strongest people generally doing 8 or 10 pounds maximum.

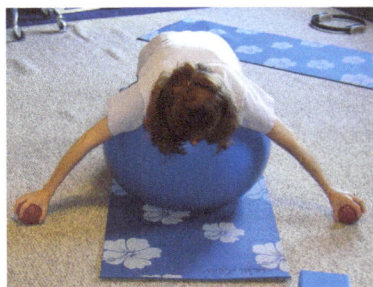

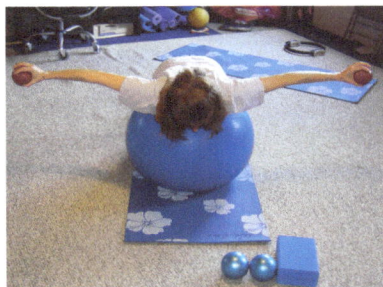

Why Strengthen Posterior Deltoid?

Posterior deltoid is actually on the upper back of the arm, and tends to get weak…that's right…because we don't use it. Rarely are people pulling things in a way that uses posterior deltoid. As with the prior two muscles, strengthen this lower shoulder muscle to reduce headaches and neck pain, forearm strain and carpal tunnel like conditions, and even out build from front and middle deltoid, chest, and bicep strengthening.

What Strengthening Posterior Deltoid Balances:

This evens out tension in neck, back, and chest muscles. Perhaps even more importantly, it takes pressure off of the Deltoids and Biceps muscles that most people strength train to look good. So, Posterior Deltoid is very much a safety muscle.

Posterior Deltoid Technical Balancing Information:

Directly, posterior deltoid strength will balance tightness found in anterior and middle deltoid fibers, which tend to be overstressed in people that pick up and carry things often or that slouch forward doing deskwork. Secondarily, posterior deltoid tone will balance proximal biceps femoris tendon, brachialis tendon, and in some clients trapezius, levator scapula, and rhomboids major and minor.

Atypical Actions

While the above 7 Safety Muscles balance the most commonly weak muscles in the body from sitting, standing, walking, running, lifting and carrying motions, there are atypical situations. One common atypical action is to carry heavy items such as bags, groceries or kids. Sometimes we carry them up hills, up or down stairs, or along extended hallways. Other time we are doing chores like vacuuming, pulling carts or luggage, or handling heavy doors as we go through airports, offices or other buidlings. Other atypical actions (or perhaps these are more typical in our computer culture) include repetitive tasks that such as assembly work, long hours at a computer, sewing, or unique movements in the surgical or dental fields.

Unique ergonomics to each job will create individualized, postural muscle patterns. While they are broadly effective, safety muscles cannot balance every activity perfectly. It is always a good idea and a safe course of action to have your postural balance evaluated by a professional. Many osteopathic physicians, chiropractors, neuromuscular therapists, physical therapists, massage therapists, or other health professionals can do a postural assessment if you ask for one. Some fitness trainers can also do a postural assessment. Ask your health professionals for more information.

Awareness & Good Form

Use good form!

Good form ensures that you are strengthening the correct muscles in each exercise. Once you are sure your form is good, you can really tell which muscles are weak based on which exercises are most challenging. Use a mirror, videotape yourself, use a trainer or physical therapist to help make sure you are using the best possible form during the exercise to get the best possible results!

Building Awareness

Doing these exercises can build your awareness. You may notice you are stronger and more upright climbing stairs or carrying bags as you get stronger and your core is more stable. Some activities and exercises will be more challenging than others. (Whatever exercise you like the least is probably the one you need the most, as you are weakest and find the exercise to be the most challenging. That's usually the way these things work.) As you grow stronger, your self-awareness helps you stay injury free and less tense. It may also make you feel more empowered and capable, so that's a big positive!

Using a professional and a mirror for help

It's always a good idea to have your form reviewed by a professional fitness trainer, exercise physiologist or physical therapist. Feel free to show them this guide to help them understand what you are doing, and want to achieve. Using a mirror by your workout area can help you use good form.

Final Results

Most participants in Safety Muscle workouts say they feel more stable, more comfortable doing activities, and less pain and discomfort when they perform these exercises 1-3 times per week. When using weights, always give your muscles 48 hours rest between exercises. This lets the muscles recover and build stronger each time.

If an exercise is really difficult to do, then you have most likely identified a weaker muscle or muscle group. Practice each exercise and notice which exercises come easily to you and which are hard to perform.

Once you have learned which muscles are weaker, you have key information to making change and relieving pain, as well as reducing your risk of injury. Focus on the weak muscles (the hardest exercises) with special diligence, as these are the ones that can create the most important changes to your posture and balance you. This in turn will help relieve pain and get you back to everyday life without the distraction of pain and poor posture. It can take 2-4 weeks to see results, so be sure to practice 3 times per week for 2-4 weeks, and see how quickly you can get a better, more pain free posture!

For further information, Questions, suggestions, or for more copies
Contact Allison Ishman
Ishman BodyCare Center, Inc.
Email ishman1@ibodycare.com **Website** www.ibodycare.com

www.ingramcontent.com/pod-product-compliance
Lightning Source LLC
Chambersburg PA
CBHW041223270326
41933CB00001B/19